HEALING IN HEELS

A Stroke Survivor's Journey
To High Heels

Dana Rivera

Table of Contents

CHAPTER 1

Living the Dream

Before June 2009, I was living my dream life. I had just celebrated my 20th wedding anniversary with my college sweetheart and was raising our four teenagers. My sons, Jake, Luke, and Nicky were playing ice hockey then, and my daughter, Sophie, was playing soccer. To say the least, there was a lot of driving involved.

Overseeing and organizing the active schedules of four children was a challenge in itself. The constant demands of being in four places at once meant that I surely had to be structured and organized, but it was what I wanted and was good at.

Before being a homemaker and mother, I never really had a passion for a career. I knew what I wanted: to marry my college sweetheart and become a mom. Aside from my "Mrs." degree in college, I also earned a Communication and Marketing Degree. We married two weeks after Rick graduated and settled in the Bay Area. I worked as a hotel concierge in the food and catering business until, six months into our marriage, the San Francisco earthquake struck. That earthquake had much to do with my decision to return to Los Angeles; I just now needed to talk Rick into moving from Northern California to Southern California. Coming from complete left field and delivering this message to him would not be easy. However, within the blink of an eye, we shared that information with my mom and dad, and we landed in Los Angeles. At the time, I was now on a new path as a wife and was soon to be a mother to one child, the second, then three, and four.

My profession was a stay-at-home mom. I loved being available for my children at any time of the day. I took great pride in being their mother and my husband's wife. I have always considered myself a traditional wife and mother. My husband was the provider, and I was his partner. We evolved into a partnership and team players. We each brought a little of how we believed we should parent to the table willingly. As a young girl, I watched my mom and how she treated my father. She followed that vision: care for the

children, make dinners, and help with home-
work. It was, in my opinion, a proper house-
wife's role.

Our dream life was a unique one. We
didn't have the traditional 6 p.m. dinners
where we all ate at the dinner table together,
sharing our stories of the day. The afternoon
pickups from school and then on to the ice
rinks sometimes went late into the evenings.
Rick and I cherished those drives because
they were an opportunity to talk with the kids,
see how their days were, and learn the latest
going on in their circle of friends. That was
one of the gifts of those teenage challenging

times: to ride in the car with your kid and hear the scoop. Yes, there were some days they didn't want to talk, so I, who doesn't have a problem talking, would always share something that was on my mind.

Of course, there were many occasions when I felt that if the kids wanted to go to an event or someone's home, and I did not have a great feeling, Rick would back me. Rick would always say to the kids, "I have to abide by your mother because when you all leave the house one day, I will be living with her." It was somewhat of a joke, but it was so true.

We were a team, and we balanced each other very well.

These were my late 20s, and I was living my dream. Then, leaning into my 30s, I matured and grew as a wife and mother, feeling confident in myself. Being fully invested in each of my children, I didn't exactly feel personal growth, but I felt a sense of growth from day-to-day experiences. I thought that was just part of the journey and living the dream. The challenge I faced in my 30s was trying to keep my children active and in line. They were young, and there were a lot of them. I was learning to balance motherhood and being a wife. I also needed to find space for myself, which was my workout routine. At that time, to get a workout in, I had to wake up at 5 a.m. to get a good 45-minute workout. I had a treadmill set up in the garage, and every morning, I set my alarm for 5 a.m. and ground it out. There was no doubt in my mind I needed this to start my day out the right way.

Surprisingly, in another blink, I turned 40. My mom was diagnosed with cancer, and at that time, it was the most enormous trauma of my life. Watching her go through that traumatic event was a devastating feeling. It was the first time death was a reality for me, other than losing my grandparents. Her illness was something very challenging for me.

I was so used to my dad fixing every-thing, and he couldn't fix this. I felt as if I was watching a horror movie. I had never really witnessed someone up close and personal to me go through a cancer journey; I didn't go to a chemo appointment or a doctor's appoint-ment because I didn't think it was the end. My perspective was, "Mom, do this so you can be better for that." It was a bit naive and out of touch.

At that time, she was given a slight chance of survivorship. Being fearful her whole life, she took her diagnosis and learned how to cope. It wasn't easy watching her go to chemo appointments. As time went by, she began to lose her hair. Watching her, step-by-step, combat her fear and uncertainty, hiring a yoga teacher to help her with some of those coping skills was huge in helping her endure. Little did I know that gift would lend itself to me.

Yoga became a place of respite for her to go deep within herself. My mother never had the tools to focus on herself and her desires because she always gave it away to those she loved. Being introduced to her yoga teacher and her deep dive into the exercise helped her with her uncertainty and anxiety about her life and what she was going through. It was amazing to witness this as her daughter; it was a real cheerleader moment.

If all your life you knew the one way to cope was pure panic and fear, and finally finding a way to help keep those emotions at bay was priceless... The yoga practice made her feel like she could learn to control her breathing and some of her body parts. It also connected to her yoga teacher, whom she believed in and respected. She was learning to trust and grow with her instructor, which was huge.

Over time, my mom got better and learned to deal with being a cancer survivor. It was clear she never could redefine herself as a survivor or help others with their uncertainty, but she did her best. I believe it was a miracle she could live 20 more years than initially predicted. That, to me, was an insane gift. She was my North Star!

My mother's journey impacted my recovery in recognizing that we are all born with resilience. Sometimes, it is not needed until a traumatic event occurs. Watching her fight each day and having faith in the things she chose to embrace helped guide me in my recovery. Sometimes with a hopeless diagnosis, you find that you embrace one another through methods of Eastern teachings and Western medicines. This, to me, was hopeful, and it showed me not to rule anything or anyone out.

CHAPTER 2

The Brush with Death

I heard a voice echo, "Miss, Miss, are you okay?" I couldn't find the words to respond as I looked down from above and saw my body lying on the floor of a clothing store—a store I had rushed into before picking up my kids from summer school.

I wanted to run into a secondhand store called Wasteland, located in the heart of Santa Monica, California. The store patrons were an eclectic mix of people: retro, rock and roll, punk rock, hippie style. Although there were no particular sounds in the store, the ambient noise from the city of Santa Monica's cars and buses permeated the space.

Every time I entered the store, I was excited to check out any vintage item I could find. It was like going on a treasure hunt and finding treasure every time. All the clothes were lined up: blouses, jeans, slacks, coats, T-shirts, and sweatshirts. There was also an area for scarves, shoes, and purses. I felt like I was in a candy store with those items.

It felt like seconds, or it could have been minutes, before I came back into my physical body and was able to find a word or two to respond to the salesperson that I thought was okay. 911 was called, and I was taken to the hospital, where, upon arrival, I was grappling with a severe headache and feeling a bit dizzy.

A neurologist examined me and thought it was a menopausal migraine. Without testing me with an MRI or CAT scan, he released me and sent me home from the hospital. At that moment, I felt relieved. Everything seemed fine except for a nagging headache. My mother was called to pick me up from the hospital. She took me home and got me settled in. My father came over to find me very incoherent and vomiting. He asked me to recite the alphabet and count. I could not do it; I was too sick and confused.

My father rushed me back to the hospital, only to see the same neurologist. When the hospital doors reopened, and he saw me return, his face was stunned, with an expression of, "Oh shit, I may have made a mistake." Doctors quickly rushed me into the MRI. I remember praying in the tightly sealed MRI tube. I was praying I wouldn't die. While I was in the MRI machine, I was praying to my husband's grandmother, Flo. Flo had a spiritual and religious way of making you feel everything would be okay. If you lost something, she would say, "Pray to St. Anthony." I loved that, and her being born on October 31st, she constantly referred to herself as a good witch.

So, as I lay in the MRI tube, I remember praying to her and asking her for guidance and direction. At that time, my husband had been reached by the police officer on duty back at the clothing store with a frantic message, "Sir, we believe your wife may have had a stroke."

Not knowing if I was going to make it or not, he rented a car, and he and my son drove five hours nonstop from Las Vegas to get to me, uncertain about what they would be faced with.

My unexpected stroke and the misdiagnosis could have been catastrophic. My emotional state at the time was pure fear and uncertainty. I was so focused on my face; was it drooping to the left side? I sure knew my arm, hand, and leg were paralyzed. There was no coldness to my hand, arm, and leg; they were like tree stumps, dead weight. My hands had a numbness to the sensation of heat or cold. I couldn't tell if something was steaming hot or freezing.

After getting out of the MRI testing, those doors flew open again, and I saw my husband and son for the first time. I was beyond scared, upset, and confused. I saw my husband's and son's faces, and it was a look of terror. The first words spoken by my husband were, "You're going to be okay, and I love you." My son's face had fright written all over it. They both came to my bedside and hugged me.

A stroke? What! How could this be? I was a perfectly fit, healthy 44-year-old. My physicality meant everything to me! I loved the gym and loved being physical. After dropping the kids off, being a gym rat was a huge part of my morning routine. I also enjoyed outdoor activities. Was that part of my life over?

ICU was next. I was so scared... I was only seeing nurses, doctors, and technicians for invasive scanners. Cameras being forced down my throat to get a clear picture of my heart only compromised the lining in my throat and esophagus. I remember the specialist coming into my room, at my bedside, while my husband watched from the background, and gently, while talking me through it, guided the camera down my throat.

I don't recall feeling anything but pure terror, and the long-term effect, I believe, is that I have a hard time sometimes swallowing or choking on food, even up to this time of my life, fourteen years later. I remember one of my nurses took to me, and I took to her. I reminded her of her mother, and she invested more than just her nurse's duties; she extended that bedside manner I needed. The hope she shed on me helped me believe, at that time, that I would get better.

Day after day, it was a dark and scary place; there were no visitors, only my husband, which I was happy about. Friends tried to get in and sneak a peek, but unbeknownst to them, they weren't allowed, period! I felt as if the doctors were putting together a football team. I had a coach, an assistant coach, and all my teammates determining my next steps.

CHAPTER 3

Uncovering the Culprit

After extensive testing, my team of doctors concluded that I had a PFO (Patent Foramen Ovale), a hole in the atrial wall of the heart affecting one in four people. I recalled the long, 20-hour flight during our beautiful 20th-anniversary trip weeks earlier. I had sat with my legs crossed the entire time, never understanding the importance of moving around on such long flights nor the benefits of compression stockings and staying hydrated. It was likely during this trip that I developed a clot, leading to Deep Vein Thrombosis (DVT).

Interestingly, most PFOs seal during the in-utero phase or shortly after birth. For some, whether it closes or remains open depends on the hole's size. The discovery of the hole only made me more proactive about getting my children checked out to see if they had a potential PFO.

From as early as six years old, I remember suffering from excruciating migraines, often finding myself in tears on the bathroom floor, trying to communicate my pain to my mom. Strangely, no doctor ever considered testing for PFO, leaving me unaware of this potential condition.

After discussing the implications of this hole with my neurologist, my biggest concern emerged: I did not want to risk another stroke. What were my options? Should I commit to taking blood thinners daily for the rest of my life? Would I need to forgo physical activities? I feared missing out on activities with my children; we had many things going on and much still to do.

On the neurologist's advice, I started consulting with cardiologists. I interviewed several, always looking for one with that crucial bedside manner that would make me feel understood and comfortable. Eventually, I found the perfect fit. There was a surgical procedure available to close the hole in my heart. Without hesitation, I was on board. Although I was still working on my physical recovery, I began to feel more like my old self with each passing day.

Six months post-stroke, my cardiologist scheduled the surgery. Eager to move forward,

I was ready to get the surgery behind me and continue rebuilding my life.

CHAPTER 4

Rebuilding from Ground Zero

My determination to return to being an independent woman, wife, and mother, which I once was, became my primary focus and way to cope with the overwhelming uncertainty and fear I felt. Something as basic as taking a shower on my own transformed into a humbling experience. I was fiercely protective of my body and its autonomy. It took a conscious mental effort to understand and accept the new routines I needed help with. My self-identity became more empowered after such a traumatic experience.

"Surrender" became my mantra, particularly when faced with the raw emotion of needing assistance for something as intimate as showering. When I returned home from the acute unit, Rick thought hiring a caregiver might be helpful. We tried it, but it was not a good fit for me. I soon realized that our longtime housekeeper, who had caregiving experience from her days before housecleaning, was the right choice. She had a pseudonym, "Virginia," from those caregiving days. So, I began calling her by that name in a light-hearted moment. It became our inside joke, reminding us that humor can be found in unexpected places. Not loving having a stranger take care of me at first, I learned to lean into my word of surrender. Another area where humor found its way in was watching more comedies; they helped lighten my emotional load.

Regaining my mobility was a significant challenge. Rick had set up outside physical therapy (PT) and occupational therapy (OT) sessions as soon as I arrived home. Our regimen included PT twice a week and OT once a week. Additionally, we instituted a morning walk ritual. Rick suggested picking a special, nearby location filled with fond memories as our destination. I chose the first neighborhood we lived in when our family began to grow; a beautiful spot overlooking the ocean. I felt invigorated to do all my therapies, PT and OT.

Starting at a vantage point where I could see and smell the vast expanse of water, I took incremental steps each day, beginning with just five. Those steps became blocks as days passed, and my balance and mobility improved.

This exercise also allowed me to process the trauma, reconnecting with a cherished past. Within a month and a half, I had worked up to two miles. My walks were therapeutic, and the scenery was the most beautiful aid in transforming my daily attitude into a positive mindset.

One day, during our walk, we ran into a gentleman who knew us from my youngest son's baseball team. Mistakenly thinking I had broken my leg; he was shocked when we told him I'd suffered a massive stroke. Reactions from the outside felt like being in a fishbowl, with everyone judging me and watching every move I made.

While I was cognitively impacted, my thoughts remained clear and my speech intact. I often describe my stroke as an earthquake— shaking and fracturing my brain, requiring time to heal and rebuild. Although my wit may have slowed down, my determination and memory never wavered. Each step towards recovery only made my resolve stronger. I read the newspaper every morning to help with my cognitive recovery.

Building confidence was, understandably, challenging. For months, I relied heavily on Rick and my family for emotional support.

If I had any regrets about my recovery journey, it would be not documenting it. Recording each milestone or journaling my feelings would have provided a tangible measure of progress. Now, I can only rely on my memory and the occasional anecdotes from acquaintances who remind me of the strength and resilience I demonstrated during that time. Initially, I felt very vulnerable sharing my story, but it built my confidence as I continued. It was important to share to help others understand that whatever issues they were dealing with, they could do so. It was all in the attitude.

CHAPTER 5

Finding Strength in Support

First, I received unwavering support from my husband, Rick. He was, and remains, my rock. Never once did he leave my side, whether I was in the ICU, the Acute Clinic, the hospital, or at home. His role as my protector and husband was both honorable and steadfast. My bond with Rick evolved into a more trusted and safer place. We knew we loved each other with all our will and might, but only when you go through the trauma do you learn what commitment and genuine love mean. We are blessed, and we know it.

From the onset of the news of my stroke, hospital visits were restricted. Many friends and family tried to see me, but access was limited. However, one evening, an individual slipped past everyone. I don't recall his name, but he mentioned he was a "friend of Bill's" and had been a patient in the same rehab unit due to a surfing accident that broke his back. His resilience and encouragement were a beacon in my darkest hours, likening him to an angel who momentarily graced my room. A stranger's visit provided hope and encouragement that things would change and evolve. It shifted my mental attitude to a growth mindset.

The visit from Bill's friend offered a fresh outlook, suggesting that if someone like him could recover, perhaps I could too. When you are engulfed in a dark abyss, the kindness of a stranger who dedicates their time to you illuminates the world's inherent goodness. It wasn't merely his stories of recovery that resonated with me but rather his insights on life after experiencing trauma. He emphasized the importance of self-compassion in the healing process. This prompted me to adopt a growth mindset, determined to pursue a complete recovery rather than resigning to a fixed mindset of "oh well, that's as good as it's going to get."

My parents were a pillar of support during this period. They visited daily. My father, who potentially saved my life by promptly getting me back to the hospital, would hold space for me every morning, offering unwavering support. I learned from this experience that loyalty, dedication, and showing up for your family are first and foremost.

Earlier, I'd mentioned my mom's journey with cancer. She lent her ear during my recovery, allowing me to vent my fears and frustrations. In a way, she saved her strength from her ordeal, bestowing it upon me when I needed it the most. She remains my North Star of inspiration.

Laurie, my older sister, was also a constant source of strength. Her presence in the hospital and during my stay in the acute unit was invaluable. Laurie, true to her role as the eldest, was always there when needed.

My younger sister, Jennifer, was prepared and proactive. She diligently cared for me, ensuring I was comfortable and well-attended. Jennifer was pivotal in getting me admitted to one of the finest acute units in town, UCLA One West Neurological.

Friends and old acquaintances showed tremendous support, dropping off groceries, preparing meals, and even chauffeuring me to therapy appointments. Admittedly, accepting help was challenging for me. But just as I had come to terms with other aspects of my new life, I surrendered to the support of those around me.

My emotional well-being fluctuated during this time. I was a scared woman, uncertain of the future. Yoga emerged as a beacon of hope. My mom had once relied on a yoga teacher during her cancer journey. Now, that same instructor, Nicole, stepped in to guide me, introducing me to yoga techniques and the power of breath to manage uncertainty and fear.

When Nicole moved away, she recommended her friend as a replacement. Though initially hesitant due to my bond with Nicole, I eventually spent ten transformative years with Venecia, practicing yoga twice a week until the COVID-19 pandemic. She became more than just a yoga instructor; she was my guide and mentor. Through yoga and her guidance, I found growth in every dimension… physically, mentally, and emotionally. She will always be a guiding light in my journey of recovery.

CHAPTER 6

Discovering a New Normal

Experiencing a stroke is like a tsunami crashing down upon you, leaving you wondering, "Where did this come from? Why is it happening?" The absence of warning signs for some makes it unexpected, and the effects lead to a complete feeling of defeat. The person I was before that moment became unrecognizable, much like the aftermath of a death. I had to grieve the loss of my former self to make way for who I would become. At times, my loss was so great that it overwhelmed me cognitively, physically, and emotionally. The only way to push through was to dig deep into my physical and mental reserves, continually reminding myself to put one foot in front of the other.

I was confronted with a changed identity: that of a stroke survivor. A recurring thought played in my mind: "My New Normal." What did that phrase truly mean? In time, I would understand its depth. Post-stroke, survivors grapple with innumerable questions:

Will I walk or talk again? Will I regain the use of my hand or arm? My foremost thought after the stroke was, am I ever going to be the same? During stroke recovery, I always found myself frustrated and lacking the tools I have today to guide me with faith.

The journey to recovery is peppered with detours and pit stops, each presenting a lesson. Gratitude emerges as a significant realization as we navigate this "new normal." It's crucial to measure progress by comparing our starting point to where we stand now. Being deep in recovery can sometimes feel like being trapped in a never-ending rabbit hole.

Finding balance as a stroke survivor is like trying to juggle all the balls at once. Balance is a word that survivors must use to feel their way through their recovery. We are thrown into so much after leaving an acute setting or hospital stay… not only do we have to create a routine of therapies, but we also have to care for our emotional loss. The roller coaster of that is difficult. As for caregivers, it's the same routine: juggle their loved ones' therapies and emotions and add to their self-care routine so they don't end up with caregiver burnout.

Amid my efforts to overcome physical limitations and in my zeal to immerse myself in therapies, I was sidelining my role as a wife and mother. Rick suggested that I gradually reintegrate into our children's daily activities.

This advice struck me profoundly. I had assumed their needs were catered to by Rick, but he believed that by sharing in their lives again, I could mentally shift from my therapeutic routines. The initial feelings of jumping back into scheduling our children's activities were pure fear. I didn't know how that would look; I was not ready, but I jumped into the deep end. This proved invaluable in my journey back to a semblance of my former self. However, I recognized that you never revert to who you once were, post-stroke.

Before this ordeal, I hadn't truly grasped the concept of resilience. Although I had given birth four times, this experience was unparalleled. I delved deeper within myself than ever before, drawing from the determination and drive that characterized my days as a dedicated gym-goer. A significant milestone in my recovery was when, on Rick's birthday, I managed to walk in high heels again. Sharing this triumph with him was a profound moment. That achievement, for me, symbolized a return to a semblance of my former self. It was an affirmation of the progress I'd made.

Independence slowly began to weave its way back into my life. Driving represents freedom for many, a means to traverse life's paths on one's terms. Bit by bit, just as I had rebuilt my walking capacity, I regained my driving skills. Initially, I drove to familiar, nearby places like the market or the dry cleaner's. The first time I got behind the wheel of my car was exciting, a bit fearful, and very conscious. The taste of that independence was exhilarating. Taking my first drive to a hockey rink was more challenging as I had to intensely control not having conversations or music--just me and the road. And if you know me, I like to talk, so that was a challenge. But once I did it, I felt like I was getting back on a bike; you don't forget. I was beyond excited to regain my independence.

In due course, I was driving my son to the ice rink again, an achievement that did not go unnoticed by the supportive moms there. My journey underscored the importance of community support. I felt an overwhelming love and support from friends, family, and acquaintances. Not everyone is fortunate enough to be surrounded by such a nurturing community, and I count it among my life's greatest blessings. Honestly, to be loved is a gift.

CHAPTER 7

Embracing Purpose

Having experienced such a traumatic event, I felt an innate need to share my story with the world. Who would have thought that at 44 years old, I'd suffer a stroke that would lead to a disability? While I was well-versed in the importance of CPR, especially having raised four children, stroke awareness was not on my radar. The general awareness about stroke is surprisingly low. Many in the community are unfamiliar with the acronym for stroke: FAST, which stands for Facial droop, Arm weakness, Speech difficulties, and Time -- emphasizing the importance of immediate medical attention. Recently, the American Heart Association introduced BEFAST, which adds Balance and Eyes to the checklist.

Even with these advances, it's startling how strokes remain the number one disability worldwide, yet public knowledge and proactive measures are not commonplace.

As I started navigating my new reality, I sought purpose beyond my old roles and identity. My unexpected encounter with a friend from the gym led to a volunteer opportunity at UCLA Ronald Reagan, the facility that was instrumental in my recovery. Here, I co-facilitated support groups in the UCLA One West Neurological Unit every Wednesday for seven years alongside another survivor. These sessions became platforms for other stroke survivors and their families, allowing them to share experiences and cope with their trauma.

The very act of sharing my story became therapeutic. It was not without its emotional toll, especially the underlying survivor's guilt. However, it became apparent that each person's stroke journey was unique, and this realization provided some solace.

Furthering my advocacy, I collaborated with the American Heart Association. A notable moment came in 2015 when I was honored to walk in the Rose Parade. Representing stroke survivors alongside individuals affected by heart disease was profoundly impactful. This advocacy led to speaking engagements and even participation in a fashion show at Stuart Weitzman in Beverly Hills. Through these experiences, my mission became clear: to raise awareness, inspire, and support others affected

by strokes.

CHAPTER 8

The Power of Purpose

As mentioned in the last chapter, I think I've discovered my purpose and wholeheartedly embraced it. In the previous 14 years, having listened to numerous survival stories, I have discerned that not everyone possesses the same drive to recover or find meaning after trauma. Depending on where the stroke occurred in the brain, it can determine a survivor's approach to recovery. A growth mindset plays a crucial role. Some settle into a passive mindset, feeling like 'this is as good as it gets', while others harness a positive mindset of giving it their all every day to reach their recovery goals.

I have collected thousands of stories over the years, all unique. The stories of fellow survivors facing worse odds than myself inspire me continually. Like most survivors, I found other's stories to be very uplifting. I started by reading the book by Dr. Jill Bolte Taylor, "My Stroke of Insight." The journey of her stroke was outside of my scope. She had to start from a true rebirth over time. I had come to learn about other personal journeys through social media, TED talks, celebrities, and exchanges at the American Heart Association events.

In my time with survivors, I have recognized that we are all born with a purpose. While some recognize it early on, it can be a continuous journey for others. An event as traumatic as a stroke can leave individuals grappling with the question: "If I can't do what I once did, what now is my purpose?" Purpose is deeply intertwined with psychological well-being, resilience, and social support, and it's indispensable for coping. Faced with a life-altering event, the once-certain path becomes murky. Some decide, "I am going to fight as hard as I can for a full recovery." Others might resign themselves to their newfound fate. Many survivors face a life of no purpose after the loss of a stroke. My job is to share that you can still have a good life if you want a purpose.

Survivors often reference a "new normal," a reality we must craft and integrate into our lives. As we navigate this journey, therapy becomes our daily rhythm. Amidst these challenges, we yearn to feel significant, believe our lives still hold meaning and direction, and contribute to society. My new normal was to accept who I am today from who I was before the stroke, meaning learning to accept that my body will forever have invisible scars from my ordeal.

Though the challenges -- be they physical, cognitive, or emotional -- might hinder us from accessing previous opportunities, new and meaningful opportunities emerge. By adopting a fresh perspective, we can identify and pursue new goals, projects, and hobbies, continually striving to offer our unique gifts to the world.

So, how do we redefine ourselves? How do we perceive our stroke as an opportunity rather than a limitation? How can we shift our narrative? Since enduring an ischemic stroke in June 2009 at 44, I've grappled with and found answers to these questions. I identified my purpose and embraced it, pivoting my focus to survival and recovery. This led me to volunteer as a stroke facilitator in the acute rehab unit, where I was once a patient. I expanded my reach to local hospitals and communities, donating my time and sharing my successful rehabilitation story. Partnering with the American Heart Association, I utilized every platform available to share my journey.

Some of those early days of volunteering were the most impactful; those early days of being allowed to be on the other side and sharing my testimony to an individual suffering through their stroke was the best feeling for me as a survivor and a volunteer. I felt as though I was like that gentleman, Bill's friend, whom I referred to in the beginning... who was to be an example and inspiration for what was to come once these patients left acute rehab. I befriended many patients and had a friendship outside the unit's cold, drab walls. I could never have met any of these individuals or family members had I not been given that volunteering opportunity.

An experience that stands out for me was meeting a woman named Linda. Linda had a stroke that left her with physical residuals. Her cognitive intake was off the charts. She was a lawyer, and so bright and cheery. I met with Linda and our group once a week for three weeks. I looked forward to seeing Linda and watching her recovery continue. We bridged a friendship and continued to speak after her acute release. Linda wanted to share her story of survival, and she and I went on to do it together. We now serve on a UCLA board for neurology patients and families. We have a virtual support group through UCLA and our monthly PFAC meetings. These board meetings try to help patients relate experiences for doctors, nurses, and social workers to make the neurology unit a better transition for patients and families. Linda has had a significant impact on me because she shared how much I inspired her to get involved in moving through her recovery.

Partnering with the American Heart Association has granted me a voice—a voice to educate, share, and serve the survivor community. I have had the privilege to connect with hundreds of survivors and their families, offering hope for a new normal. Fourteen years post-stroke, I've harnessed my pain, which gave it purpose and turned it into something beautiful. I fervently hope my fellow stroke survivors can do the same.

CHAPTER 9

A Journey of Hope and Reflection

Every year on June 29th, I take a moment to reflect on my journey since suffering a massive stroke at the age of 44. Each anniversary, I celebrate and ponder how blessed I am: firstly, to have survived; secondly, to have experienced a successful recovery; and lastly, to provide hope for those just beginning their paths to recovery. Hope was essential for me; it was a daily source of strength. Without hope and faith, I might not have navigated the most challenging times of my recovery.

When you are open to viewing recovery as an opportunity to reinvent yourself, it allows you to start with a blank canvas and paint a whole new picture filled with excitement and possibility. An invaluable lesson from my journey was learning the essence of "patience." With this type of recovery, it truly becomes a "one day at a time" mantra. Patience is a hard practice to learn. You must work on it daily.

It requires me to go deep within my comfort zone and not spiral out of control. I do this by reading my affirmations or just a great quote from someone. I find that my set-backs are sometimes more of my old habits of thinking and processing. When I feel those old habits simmering within myself, I must acknowledge them first so I can put a lid on them. This allows me to draw from the new strategies that I've learned to carry through my day.

I have also seen tremendous personal growth, immersing myself in a new environ-ment. Recognizing stroke as a neurological event, I challenged myself to collaborate with hospitals and create support groups. These groups act as crucial resources, offering hope, encouragement, and support… particularly for caregivers of stroke survivors. Providing a non-judgmental space for them to share their experiences is essential.

Feeling a desire to contribute even more within the neurological community, I discovered the Acquired Brain Injury program at Santa Monica Community College, which aids students with various neurological issues. Pitching my idea for a stroke support group to the college's decision-makers took about two years, but my persistence paid off. Offering support to these students remains a point of pride for me. It evolved into a wellness program, providing students with an environment to discuss daily challenges and accomplishments. Such spaces counteract feelings of isolation, a common issue for many. I made these groups come to fruition through pure work, never taking no for an answer and seeing it as a persistent mission and vision. Having empathy and compassion lends me emotional tolerance for all survivor stories. My gratitude for my recovery helps me hold everyone's stories with grace.

As with any professional who works with individuals, it is difficult not to take on others' pain, struggles, or uncertainty. I have always been empathetic, and realizing others have a more difficult life or circumstances was made clear as I continued my work through the support setting. I always want my members to know there is light, and to continue to follow the light so they can use it like their sector to see beauty in the trauma, and the gifts they (and I) have been given from our trauma to keep carrying them on through.

I joined a program called Kandu Health, which offers personalized support to stroke survivors. In my role as a Kandu Ambassador,

I co-facilitate sessions alongside another facilitator and a Kandu navigator. Looking ahead, I am eager to embark on new ventures. I'm considering launching a podcast and exploring more motivational speaking opportunities to raise awareness about heart disease and the importance of self-advocacy. My podcast will include interviews with survivors. Every survivor carries a chance to spread hope, encouragement, and inspiration, that maybe someone else is lacking or can't find within themselves. It can take just one flicker of a word or a complete conversation to connect and reframe how a survivor thinks about their recovery.

It's vital for me not to become compla

cent. If I do, my growth and mission to inspire will stagnate. I believe in continuously sharing and emphasizing the importance of personal health and advocacy. After all, investing in our-selves is the key to becoming the best versions of ourselves. Health always comes first!

CHAPTER 10

The Gift of Faith

One of the personal gifts my husband instilled in me was his unwavering faith. I'm not referring to the faith of a religious or spiritual kind but a foundational belief that irrespective of challenges, things will find a way to work out. From the early days of starting our family, we

constantly said, "We have to have faith," espe
cially when we faced hurdles.

The aftermath of the stroke was overwhelming, particularly grappling with the disability that affected my left side-- my hand, arm,
and leg. Beyond this, the most immediate fear
was of the stroke being fatal. However, a transformative moment occurred during a solitary
night in the ICU. I focused intently, willing my
left leg to lift, and to my surprise, it did! That
movement, however minor, occurring at 3 am,
became a monumental beacon of hope for me.
Sharing this triumph with my neurologist the
following day reinforced my renewed spirit.

When I was able to lift my leg up from the hospital bed, it was a sign to keep going, to believe I can, and will, make that comeback. Faith.

Annually, on the anniversary of my stroke, I engage in introspection. I've made it a tradition to share my reflections and lessons on social media. This year's message centered on "TIME," emphasizing that time is our most precious asset and urging its judicious investment.

While we can control certain lifestyle choices to reduce stroke risks, like high blood pressure or smoking, there are unpredictable elements, such as unknown genetic factors, which was my case. The lesson is twofold: exert control where possible and embrace acceptance where it is not.

Recovery from a stroke isn't a sprint but a marathon, a progression taken one day at a time. Using past milestones as reference points reminds us how far we have traveled. Adopting the practice of living in the present, aided by daily mantras, helps me overcome my inherent tendency to worry.

In retrospect, I wish I had meticulously documented my recovery journey, capturing both my emotions and physical progress on video. Relying primarily on memory means some details blur, but occasionally, encounters with acquaintances bring forgotten aspects to light. One particularly touching memory was my decision to revisit the acute unit's therapists, at six months post-stroke. Walking into that space, observing their reactions to my progress, and particularly showcasing my regained ability to walk confidently in heels was not just a testament to my journey but a reaffirmation of the power of hope, faith, and unwavering effort.

CHAPTER 11

Living a Life of Purpose

Recovery is a winding journey, fraught with de-tours and setbacks; it is far from a straight path. Although I have touched upon the concept of purpose in previous chapters, I have realized that one does not discover it instantly. As a stroke survivor, my mission evolved into seek-ing an authentic life -- a life original to me,

achieved through discipline and intention. Be
fore the stroke, my life was primarily about
raising my family. They were my everything,
and the hope of returning to that role, wholly
intact, drove me toward a balanced, committed
life.

Every stroke survivor carries a unique
story. Just as no two fingerprints are identical,
every survivor faces the challenge of redefining
who they are, separate from their past selves.
Over my fourteen years of facilitating support
groups, I've observed that many survivors have
'Type A' personalities. While there is no guar-
antee that survivors will regain all they once

had, striving relentlessly toward recovery is crucial.

My ambition was to create something that instills hope and offers validation. Embracing change has been a significant facet of my journey, and much of my personal growth has sprouted from my newfound purpose. It is important to note that not every survivor will find a distinct purpose, especially since many are engrossed in the rigorous physical and mental recovery process. Grief sometimes remains. However, confronting that grief, accepting it, and navigating through it can become a guiding purpose for many.

Navigating life after a significant trauma requires resilience and a strong support system. It's crucial to surround oneself with individuals who echo your aspirations; often, those connections help discover and solidify one's purpose. I was fortunate to connect with many survivors, caregivers, and advocates who, through shared experiences, shaped my vision for the future.

Over time, I have come to understand that having a purpose is not trying to reach a final destination but an ongoing journey. It's about continuous evolution, learning, and growth. Living a life of purpose is akin to planting a tree; it may start as a tiny sapling, but with care, patience, and nurturing, it grows strong, offering shade and fruits to those around it.

FROM THE AUTHOR'S HEART

AFTERWORD

Heels were an important part of who I was, and I sure loved my wedges. The thought of never being able to walk in those wedges was another layer I had to think of peeling away at my former self. I loved a good wedge shoe, and when I was finally able put my left foot back into one of my wedges, I felt a burst of joy. It was exhilarating to walk step by step in those heels as they guided me into a happy place of something and someone familiar. I cannot speak for other women, but I felt it was a beautiful thing to strut down a street in a great pair of jeans and a better pair of heels. Remembering when I was hospitalized and raised my left leg again gave me that a ray of hope and possibility. To this day, I look at heels as a special accessory to my outfit. I wear my heels with a proud smile on my face... strutting one step at a time.

Made in the USA
Columbia, SC
08 August 2024

40188874R00054